Cantaloupe Salmonella Outbreak

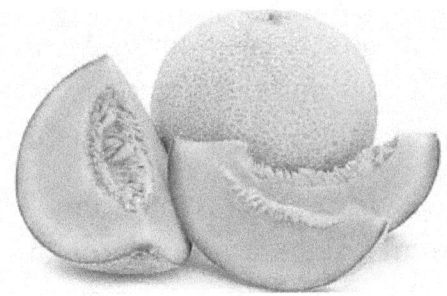

Tracing the Tragedy, Ongoing Consequences and Preventive Measures Against Contamination

Carole J. Powell

Table of Contents

Introduction

In the landscape of food safety, there emerges a silent yet potent threat—one that disrupts our confidence in the produce aisle, challenges our understanding of health, and raises profound concerns about the safety of what we consume daily.

The **Cantaloupe Salmonella Outbreak** is not just a singular event but a wake-up call to a larger reality: the vulnerability lurking within our food chain. It's a cautionary tale that transcends the confines of a mere outbreak—it's a narrative entwined with microbiology, the interplay of bacteria and food, and the intricacies of our health.

In this riveting journey, we explore a haunting narrative that unfolded with the innocent backdrop of the produce section, where cantaloupes—succulent, inviting, and seemingly harmless—became the carriers of a stealthy menace. The outbreak, sparked by contaminated fruit, exposed hundreds to the menacing grasp of Salmonella, leaving behind a trail of illness, hospitalizations, and even tragedy.

But this tale extends far beyond the outbreak itself. It delves deep into the microscopic world of bacteria, the historical arras of cantaloupes, and the intricate processes behind cultivation, distribution, and consumption. It's a story that unearths the realities of foodborne illnesses, the strains of Salmonella, and the grave repercussions they bear on public health.

As your guide through this web of knowledge and awareness, I invite you not only to witness the tale of the

Cantaloupe Salmonella Outbreak but to embark on a transformative journey. This book is not merely about an isolated incident—it's a testament to the complexities of food safety, the rich heritage of cantaloupes, and the imperative need for informed decisions.

I stand as an advocate for knowledge, empowerment, and health. My aim is to equip you with insights, understanding, and actionable steps—empowering you to make informed choices, safeguard your well-being, and navigate the intricacies of food safety in a world teeming with culinary delights.

Throughout these pages, we'll unravel the mysteries behind Salmonella, decode the nuances of cantaloupes, and explore the intricate web that connects our food from farm to table. We'll journey into the microscopic realms and culinary landscapes, shedding light on the preventive measures, health implications, and culinary treasures entwined within this narrative.

This book is your gateway to a world where knowledge combats fear, awareness fosters empowerment, and understanding transforms into action. Join me as we uncover the nuances of the Cantaloupe Salmonella Outbreak, navigating the complexities, unraveling the mysteries, and igniting a pursuit for safer, more informed choices.

Chapter 1

The severity and impact of foodborne illnesses

Foodborne illnesses are a serious and widespread concern impacting the health of people worldwide. These illnesses are caused by harmful microorganisms like bacteria, viruses, parasites, or even toxic substances such as heavy metals found in the food we consume. Can you imagine that the very food we rely on for sustenance can sometimes carry such hidden dangers?

The World Health Organization (WHO) highlights that there are more than 200 known diseases directly linked to consuming contaminated food. These diseases aren't just a small problem – they contribute significantly to the global burden of sickness and death. Shockingly, every year, around 600 million cases of foodborne diseases crop up across the globe, and sadly, approximately 420,000 people lose their lives due to these illnesses. These numbers are staggering and emphasize the urgency of addressing food safety on a global scale.

Certain groups of people face higher risks when it comes to these illnesses. Children younger than 5 years old and older adults aged 65 years and above are particularly vulnerable. Their immune systems might not be as strong, making them more susceptible to getting seriously sick from contaminated food. For them, a seemingly harmless meal could lead to severe health issues or, in tragic cases, even death.

It's crucial for everyone to understand the importance of food safety measures. Simple steps like proper hygiene during food preparation, thorough cooking of food, safe storage, and avoiding cross-contamination can significantly reduce the risk of falling ill from foodborne pathogens. Education and awareness about safe food handling practices are essential for safeguarding health.

By raising awareness about these risks and promoting safe food practices, we can collectively work towards reducing the incidence of foodborne illnesses, protecting vulnerable populations, and ensuring that the food we consume is not just tasty but also safe and healthy for all.

Preview of the Cantaloupe Salmonella Outbreak case

The Cantaloupe Salmonella Outbreak has left a significant impact on both the United States and Canada, affecting numerous individuals. This outbreak was traced back to contaminated cantaloupes, carrying the dangerous salmonella bacteria. The most recent count, as of December 16, 2023, reports a staggering 129 cases of illness and sadly, six deaths across both countries due to this outbreak.

Salmonella poisoning brings along a range of distressing symptoms including diarrhea, fever, stomach cramps, nausea, vomiting, and headaches. These symptoms can be quite uncomfortable and can last for several days, disrupting daily life and causing immense discomfort for those affected. While investigations are ongoing, the exact source of the contamination that led to this outbreak remains unknown.

Foodborne illnesses like salmonella poisoning aren't just short-lived troubles. They can have severe, long-lasting effects on our health. Beyond the immediate discomfort, these illnesses may cause lasting health issues such as kidney failure, chronic arthritis, and even damage to the brain and nerves. This isn't just about feeling unwell for a few days; it can have a lasting impact on a person's overall well-being. Moreover, these illnesses bring with them additional problems like lost productivity, medical bills, premature deaths, and immense pain and suffering. People who are more vulnerable, like children, pregnant or post-partum women, elderly individuals, and those with weakened immune systems, face a higher risk of severe illness due to these contaminated foods.

Preventing these illnesses is crucial, and there are steps everyone can take to minimize the risk. Following food safety guidelines is essential. Avoiding consumption of products that have been recalled due to contamination is a simple yet vital step to safeguard oneself from falling ill. Additionally, thoroughly washing all fruits and vegetables before consuming them is highly recommended. This small action significantly reduces the risk of getting sick from harmful bacteria lingering on the produce.

The Centers for Disease Control and Prevention (CDC) are actively collaborating with state and local health departments, along with the Food and Drug Administration (FDA), and other partners to dig deep into this outbreak. Their collective aim is not only to understand how this contamination happened but also to prevent similar outbreaks from occurring in the future. This collaborative effort is crucial in safeguarding public health and ensuring that such incidents are minimized or avoided altogether.

By working together and being vigilant about food safety practices, we can significantly reduce the chances of experiencing the devastating impacts of foodborne illnesses like the Cantaloupe Salmonella Outbreak. It's not just about reacting to outbreaks but also about taking proactive steps to protect ourselves and our communities from such health hazards.

Chapter 2

Understanding Salmonella

What is Salmonella

Salmonella is a sneaky germ that hangs out in the tummies of both people and animals. It's a type of bacteria that can make us really sick if we eat or drink something that's been infected with it. These bacteria have a rod-like shape when seen under a super-powerful microscope, and they belong to a big family called **Enterobacteriaceae.**

When these little bacteria get into our bodies, they can cause a bunch of health issues known as salmonellosis. It's not a fun experience! Imagine having a really bad stomach ache, feeling super queasy, having a fever, and dealing with frequent trips to the bathroom—all because these tiny bacteria are causing trouble inside us.

The tricky part about Salmonella is that we often can't see it, taste it, or smell it in our food or water. So, if it's lurking in something we eat or drink, it can cause a lot of harm without us even knowing it's there. That's why it's important to make sure the food we eat is prepared safely and cooked properly to kill off these harmful bacteria and keep us healthy.

Characteristics of Salmonella

Salmonella bacteria are rod-shaped, gram-negative, facultatively anaerobic bacteria that are approximately 2-5 micrometers in length and 0.7-1.5 micrometers in diameter. They are motile, with peritrichous flagella that allow them to move through liquid environments. Salmonella bacteria are capable of surviving in a wide range of environments, including soil, water, and food products. There are over 2,500 serotypes of Salmonella, which are classified based on their antigenic properties.

Salmonella bacteria: morphology and behavior

Picture Salmonella bacteria as these tiny, rod-shaped creatures that are very, very small—around 2 to 5 micrometers long and 0.7 to 1.5 micrometers wide. They're so tiny that you need a special microscope to see them! These bacteria are a bit like us—they can survive with or without oxygen, which is what "facultatively anaerobic" means. It's like saying they're flexible about where they live; they're comfortable in different environments.

Now, these Salmonella bacteria are movers! They've these tiny hair-like things called flagella all around their bodies. It's like they've little tails that help them swim around, especially in liquids. That's how they move through stuff like water and other liquids.

These bacteria are also tough survivors. They can live in many places—imagine hanging out in soil, water, and even in different types of food. They're like the ultimate adventurers, going anywhere they can find a cozy spot to settle in.

So, even though they're super tiny and might seem harmless because we can't see them, these Salmonella bacteria are quite resourceful in finding their way into various places and sticking around. That's why it's crucial to handle food properly and cook it thoroughly to make sure we keep these sneaky bacteria out of our meals and stay healthy.

Different types of Salmonella and their effects on humans.

Think of Salmonella like having a big family with lots of cousins! There are more than 2,500 types, or what we call "serotypes," of Salmonella. These types are sorted out based on their special features that help us recognize them. But among this big family, two cousins—Salmonella Typhimurium and Salmonella Enteritidis—are the troublemakers when it comes to making humans sick.

When these cousins, Typhimurium and Enteritidis, sneak into our bodies through contaminated food or water, they can cause quite a ruckus! They bring along a range of unpleasant symptoms like a really upset tummy with diarrhea, high fever, stomach cramps that hurt a lot, and sometimes throwing up. Imagine feeling really sick and uncomfortable—all because of these sneaky bacteria.

In serious cases, these Salmonella infections can land us in the hospital because our bodies can get severely dehydrated from all the diarrhea and vomiting. And in very rare and extreme situations, it can even lead to someone passing away, though that's really uncommon.

It's like these Salmonella cousins come to our bodies and start a not-so-fun party that we definitely don't want to attend. So, it's crucial to make sure we handle and cook our food properly to keep these troublemaking bacteria out of our meals. By doing this, we can avoid their unwanted visits and keep ourselves healthy and feeling good.

Historical background and notable outbreaks

Salmonella was first identified by an American scientist named Daniel E. Salmon in 1885. Since then, there have been many notable outbreaks of salmonella infection around the world.

Like in the United States in 1985, there was a big issue when milk from just one farm in Illinois had these germs. It made more than 16,000 people very sick. That's a lot of folks dealing with bad stomach aches and feeling really unwell because of this contaminated milk.

Then in 2010, there was another problem. Eggs from a farm in Iowa had these same germs, and it made over 1,900 people sick after eating those eggs. It was like these germs made a lot of people feel really bad because the eggs weren't safe to eat.

Jumping ahead to more recent times, in 2023, there was a big outbreak again. This time, it was because of cantaloupes that had these germs in them. Sadly, by December 16, 2023, at least 129 people got sick, and six people passed away in Canada and the United States because of these contaminated cantaloupes. It was a really sad and worrying time.

The hard part is that even though we know these outbreaks happened, sometimes it's tough to find out exactly where the germs came from. It's like trying to solve a mystery! Investigators are still trying to figure out how these germs got into the food, especially in the case of the Cantaloupe Salmonella Outbreak.

These stories show how these sneaky germs, Salmonella, can cause big problems and make lots of people sick. That's why it's super important to handle our food carefully, cook it properly, and make sure it's safe to eat. By doing this, we can help stop these kinds of outbreaks and keep everyone healthy and feeling good.

Chapter 3

Origins of the Outbreak

People in the United States and Canada got really worried because of something called the **Cantaloupe Salmonella Outbreak**. This outbreak became a huge problem for everyone's health.

So, what really happened? Well, it's like a detective story! Investigators began looking for clues to understand where this outbreak started. They traced it back to when the first reports came in. People started feeling sick after eating cantaloupes. The detectives—these are actually health experts—worked hard to find out which cantaloupes were making people sick.

They found out that some of these tasty cantaloupes were carrying something really bad—Salmonella germs! These sneaky germs got into the cantaloupes somehow, and when people ate them, they got really sick. It was like a puzzle to figure out how these germs got into the fruit.

There were different things that could have caused the contamination, like maybe dirty water used in the fields where the cantaloupes grew, or maybe the way they were handled and stored after being picked. Investigators checked all these possibilities to find out how these germs got into the cantaloupes.

When they found out about this problem, people and health experts took quick action! They wanted to stop more people from getting sick, so they worked hard to remove the contaminated cantaloupes from stores. It was like a big effort to stop these bad cantaloupes from reaching more people and causing more sickness.

Tracing the Genesis of the Cantaloupe Salmonella Outbreak

The Cantaloupe Salmonella Outbreak was first identified in November 2023, when the Centers for Disease Control and Prevention (CDC) issued a warning about the outbreak. The CDC reported that the outbreak was linked to cantaloupes that were contaminated with salmonella. The exact source of the contamination was not immediately known, and an investigation was launched to determine the origin of the outbreak.

Initial reports and identification of contaminated cantaloupes.

In the early days of the Cantaloupe Salmonella Outbreak, troubling reports surfaced from people who fell ill after enjoying these sweet melons. The Centers for Disease Control and Prevention (CDC) stepped into action, launching an investigation to uncover the truth behind this growing health concern. They reached out to those affected, gathering crucial details about their experiences.

Through these conversations, a pattern emerged—cantaloupes were at the heart of this distressing situation. It was like fitting puzzle pieces together. The stories from those who fell sick pointed to these delightful fruits as the likely culprits.

But that wasn't the end of the detective work. The CDC collaborated closely with local health groups to dig deeper. Their goal was to pinpoint the specific brands of cantaloupes that carried this harmful salmonella. These health workers combed through information to crack the case wide open.

Their investigation spotlighted two particular brands—Malichita and Rudy. These cantaloupes turned out to be carriers of the dangerous salmonella bacteria. And what made it scarier was that these contaminated fruits has been distributed far and wide, spreading across both the United States and Canada.

It was like discovering the key players in a mystery—a big breakthrough in understanding where these harmful fruits came from. This discovery not only connected the dots but also sounded a warning, urging caution for anyone who might have bought these brands. The identification of these contaminated cantaloupes was a pivotal step towards containing the outbreak and protecting more people from falling ill.

Factors contributing to contamination

The exact reasons behind how the cantaloupes got contaminated are still a bit of a mystery. But there are some important things to consider that might have been involved in causing this outbreak.

Firstly, let's talk about where these cantaloupes come from—soil! Cantaloupes grow in the ground, and if the soil they grow in has salmonella in it, then the cantaloupes could pick up these harmful germs. It's like if you're playing outside and accidentally get dirt on your hands, right? The soil can sometimes have bad stuff in it, and that might have happened with these fruits.

Then there's the way these melons were handled during harvest time and when they were being packed up for stores. If the people picking the cantaloupes or packing them didn't follow good cleanliness rules, like washing their hands or making sure the tools they used were clean, the cantaloupes could have picked up germs along the way. It's like if someone is cooking and forgets to wash their hands before touching the food—they could pass on germs without knowing.

These might seem like small things, but when it comes to food safety, even the tiniest slip-ups can cause big problems. It's kind of like a chain reaction; if one step isn't done right, it can affect the whole process.

Early responses and containment efforts

The CDC and the Food and Drug Administration (FDA) responded quickly to the Cantaloupe Salmonella Outbreak. The FDA issued a recall of all cantaloupes that were linked to the outbreak, and the CDC advised people to avoid eating cantaloupes until the source of the outbreak was identified.

The FDA and the CDC worked with state and local health departments to investigate the outbreak and identify the source of the contamination. The FDA conducted inspections of the farms and packing facilities that were associated with the contaminated cantaloupes, and the CDC collected samples of the cantaloupes for testing.

The FDA and the CDC also worked with retailers and distributors to remove the contaminated cantaloupes from the market. The FDA issued a recall of all cantaloupes that were linked to the outbreak, and the CDC advised people to avoid eating cantaloupes until the source of the outbreak was identified.

The Cantaloupe Salmonella Outbreak was a significant public health concern in the United States and Canada. The outbreak was traced to contaminated cantaloupes, and the FDA and the CDC responded quickly to contain the outbreak.

Though the exact reasons behind the cantaloupe contamination remain elusive, it's evident that proper hygiene practices play a crucial role in preventing future outbreaks. It's like learning from a tough lesson—the importance of cleanliness in ensuring our food is safe.

Simple acts like washing hands and keeping things clean can make a huge difference in keeping harmful germs away from our fruits and our bodies.

In the end, the Cantaloupe Salmonella Outbreak was a stark reminder of the delicate balance between food safety and public health. The FDA and CDC's rapid response highlighted the critical need for vigilance and collaboration in safeguarding our well-being. It's a story of caution, collaboration, and the collective efforts aimed at protecting everyone from the hidden dangers that might lurk in our food.

Chapter 4

Contaminated Cantaloupes: A Closer Look.

Those juicy fruits we all love, somehow turned into carriers of a sneaky germ called Salmonella. But how did these innocent fruits become unsafe to eat?

It starts where these melons grow—the farms. Sometimes, the soil where the cantaloupes grow might have Salmonella in it. If the soil was contaminated, the germs might've gotten into the melons as they were growing.

Then, when it's time to pick these fruits, things like how they're handled or packed could have played a part. If the folks picking or packing the cantaloupes didn't wash their hands or use clean tools, they could've passed on the germs without knowing.

Farming and harvesting practices linked to contamination

The way cantaloupes are grown and harvested can play a significant role in the spread of salmonella. For example, if the water used for irrigation or washing the fruits is contaminated, it can spread the germs onto the cantaloupes. Similarly, if the harvesting tools or containers are dirty, they can cause contamination as well.

In fact, the FDA found that field contamination was a significant factor in the Cantaloupe Salmonella Outbreak. The FDA conducted an extensive investigation of cantaloupe and watermelon growing operations at Chamberlain Farms in Owensville, Indiana, after an initial inspection found one of the outbreak strains in the packing area, two outbreak strains from cantaloupes collected from the field, and one outbreak strain from a watermelon growing area.

It is essential to follow proper hygiene practices during the growing and harvesting of cantaloupes to prevent contamination. This includes using clean water for irrigation and washing, ensuring that harvesting tools and containers are clean, and following proper sanitation practices. By following these practices, we can help prevent future outbreaks of salmonella contamination in cantaloupes.

Environmental factors facilitating bacterial growth.

Environmental factors can play a significant role in the growth and spread of salmonella on cantaloupes. Salmonella bacteria thrive in warm, moist environments, and if the weather or temperature is just right, they can grow and multiply on the cantaloupes.

In addition to temperature, other environmental factors that can facilitate bacterial growth include humidity, soil conditions, and the presence of other microorganisms.

Identifying vulnerable points in the supply chain.

The journey of cantaloupes from farms to stores is like a winding road with various stops along the way. At each of these stops, something could have gone amiss, leading to the risk of contamination and making these fruits potentially unsafe to eat. Understanding these vulnerable points in the supply chain is key to uncovering the roots of contamination.

Farming Practices: Starting at the farms, during the growth and harvesting phases, practices like irrigation with contaminated water, improper handling by farmworkers, or the use of unclean harvesting tools could introduce germs to the cantaloupes.

Packing and Processing: As the fruits are sorted, packed, and processed, any oversight in hygiene practices at these facilities might contribute to contamination. If the environment isn't kept clean or if the equipment used isn't sanitized properly, it can pose a risk.

Transportation: Once packed, the cantaloupes embark on a journey. During transportation, if the vehicles aren't sanitized or if the fruits come into contact with unclean surfaces, it could lead to contamination. Temperature changes during transit might also influence bacterial growth.

Storage Facilities: Upon arrival at warehouses or storage units, the conditions in which the cantaloupes are stored matter. Improper temperature controls or storage alongside contaminated items could increase the risk of contamination.

Retail Handling: At stores, the way cantaloupes are displayed or handled can be crucial. If the store environment isn't clean, or if there's a mix-up with other contaminated produce, the risk of cross-contamination rises.

Consumer Practices: Even at home, improper washing or handling of cantaloupes could contribute to the risk. If people don't wash the fruits before cutting into them or use utensils that aren't clean, it could spread germs.

Identifying these vulnerable points is like creating a roadmap of possible trouble spots. Each step in this journey from farm to fork presents an opportunity for contamination. Pinpointing these weak links in the chain helps in devising strategies to ensure proper safety measures are implemented at every stage. It's about reinforcing hygiene protocols, improving handling practices, and maintaining clean environments to reduce the risks of contamination and keep our food supply safe.

Chapter 5

Impact and Affected Population

The Cantaloupe Salmonella Outbreak has had a significant impact on public health in the United States and Canada. In this chapter, we'll explore the toll of the outbreak on public health and affected demographics, provide a statistical breakdown of the number of affected individuals and regions, discuss case studies of affected individuals and communities, and examine the health complications and long-term implications of the outbreak.

As of December 6, 2023, the alarming statistics revealed a staggering count—230 reported cases of salmonella infection were directly linked to this outbreak. Among these cases, a chilling 96 people had to be hospitalized due to the severity of their symptoms, highlighting the seriousness of the situation. To compound the devastation, this outbreak led to the heartbreaking loss of three precious lives, a grim reminder of the potency of foodborne illnesses.

What's particularly concerning is that this outbreak did not discriminate—it affected people across various age groups. However, the impact was especially severe among the more vulnerable sections of the population. Children under the age of 5 and elderly adults over 65 faced a higher risk of enduring severe symptoms due to their weaker immune systems. These age groups are more susceptible to falling seriously ill when exposed to harmful bacteria like Salmonella.

The toll on public health wasn't merely about numbers; it was about individuals—mothers, fathers, sons, and daughters—who fell victim to the consequences of consuming contaminated cantaloupes. Families faced the anguish of seeing their loved ones suffer, some enduring the distressing ordeal of hospitalization, while others mourned the unimaginable loss of cherished lives.

This outbreak's impact reverberated across communities, triggering concerns about food safety and the vulnerability of certain groups to foodborne illnesses. It underscored the importance of stringent measures to safeguard food and protect public health. As the outbreak unfolded, it stood as a somber reminder of the critical need for heightened vigilance in ensuring the safety of our food supply.

Health complications and long-term implications

Salmonella infection, a distressing consequence of consuming contaminated food like the tainted cantaloupes, can set off a host of distressing symptoms that wreak havoc on the body. Imagine your body's defense system encountering a sneaky invader—it's like an unwelcome guest causing chaos within.

The symptoms of this infection are no light matter—diarrhea, fever, abdominal cramps, and vomiting. It's akin to your body going into a full-scale battle mode, trying to flush out these harmful bacteria. But for some unfortunate souls, it can get worse. Severe cases can lead to hospitalization—

a daunting prospect for anyone battling the aftermath of consuming contaminated food. Dehydration can set in, adding to the physical distress, and in the most tragic circumstances, it can even result in death. It's like your body facing a relentless assault, struggling to fight off the effects of this harmful bacteria.

While many recover from salmonella infection without enduring long-term effects, some face a lingering aftermath. Imagine the infection as a shadow—after it's seemingly gone, it might leave behind traces of trouble. For some, it's reactive arthritis—an unwelcome companion that causes joint pain and swelling. It's like an aftermath, a reminder of the havoc the infection caused in the body, particularly targeting the joints, making even the simplest movements a painful ordeal.

These long-term effects aren't just physical—they're emotional and mental too. Imagine the strain on someone who battles daily joint pain, a constant reminder of the infection's aftermath. It's not just about the immediate illness; it's about the long road to recovery, both physically and emotionally, for those who endure these lingering effects.

Chapter 6

Symptoms of Salmonella Poisoning

Salmonella poisoning is like an unwelcome guest that brings along a host of distressing symptoms, making you feel quite under the weather. It's crucial to recognize these signs as they indicate that something might not be right within your body.

Early Signs and Progression of the Illness

At the onset, symptoms often start subtly, creeping in like uninvited guests. You might notice things like an upset stomach, abdominal cramps, or a general feeling of being unwell. As time passes, these symptoms can worsen, escalating to fever, diarrhea, and vomiting. It's like your body trying to battle an unseen enemy, and these symptoms are its way of signaling that something is off.

Variations in symptoms among different demographics

Interestingly, the way salmonella manifests itself can differ among various groups of people. For some, especially young children and elderly individuals, the symptoms might be more severe. Kids might experience more pronounced gastrointestinal issues, while older adults might face challenges with dehydration or more intense abdominal discomfort. It's like this unwanted visitor affecting each person in a slightly different way, making it crucial to pay attention to individual experiences.

Steps to Differentiate Salmonella from Other Illnesses

Distinguishing salmonella from other illnesses can be tricky since its symptoms can resemble those of various stomach bugs or food-related issues. However, certain clues might help set it apart. The timing—especially if symptoms start after consuming certain foods—could be a clue. Also, the duration and severity of symptoms, along with any possible known exposure to contaminated food, can be key factors to consider.

Understanding these symptoms is crucial. It's like learning to decipher your body's distress signals, enabling you to recognize when something isn't quite right. This knowledge empowers you to take necessary steps, seek appropriate medical attention, and also helps in preventing the spread of illness to others. Being vigilant about these symptoms aids in swift identification and treatment, ensuring a speedier recovery.

Chapter 7

Responding to Suspected Exposure

Discovering or suspecting exposure to Salmonella warrants prompt action. Begin by immediately avoiding the suspected food or source of contamination. Hygiene is crucial—wash your hands thoroughly with soap and water after handling potentially contaminated items, and ensure surfaces are cleaned to prevent the spread of germs.

Seeking medical attention: when and how

If you're unsure whether your symptoms warrant medical attention, it's always a good idea to consult your healthcare provider. Reach out if your symptoms don't improve after a few days, if they worsen, or if you're concerned about your well-being. For vulnerable groups like young children, older adults, pregnant individuals, or those with weakened immune systems, it's essential to err on the side of caution and seek medical advice early in the course of illness.

How to Seek Medical Attention: Contact your healthcare provider's office or clinic and describe your symptoms, specifying your concerns regarding potential Salmonella exposure. They might advise you to come in for an evaluation, provide guidance over the phone, or direct you to the appropriate healthcare facility for further assessment and treatment.

Importance of Medical Evaluation: While many cases of Salmonella resolve without medical intervention, certain situations might require medical evaluation. Seeking medical attention can ensure a proper diagnosis, rule out other potential causes, and, if necessary, receive treatment such as fluid replacement therapy for dehydration or antibiotics in severe cases.

Remember, the goal of seeking medical attention is not just to address the current symptoms but also to prevent potential complications and ensure your well-being. Your healthcare provider can offer tailored guidance based on your individual circumstances and provide the necessary support for a speedy recovery.

Self-care measures and home remedies for mild cases

Preventing the spread of Salmonella within your household is essential. Be vigilant about hygiene—wash hands thoroughly, especially before handling food or after using the bathroom.

Thorough Handwashing: Start with the basics—washing hands diligently. Scrub your hands with soap and water for at least 20 seconds before handling food, after using the restroom, or after any activities that might involve potential contamination.

Surface Disinfection: Regularly clean and disinfect surfaces that frequently come into contact with food or potentially contaminated items. Use hot, soapy water to clean countertops, cutting boards, utensils, and kitchen tools. Disinfect these surfaces using a diluted bleach solution or a disinfectant spray to ensure thorough sanitation.

Safe Food Handling:

Separation of Raw and Ready-to-Eat Foods: Practice caution while handling raw foods, particularly meats, poultry, and seafood. Keep them separate from ready-to-eat foods like fruits, vegetables, and cooked items to prevent cross-contamination. Use separate cutting boards and utensils for raw and cooked foods.

Cooking Temperatures: Cooking foods, especially meat products, to the appropriate temperatures is crucial in killing harmful bacteria like Salmonella. Use a food thermometer to ensure meats reach their recommended internal temperature. For instance, poultry should reach 165°F (73.9°C), ground beef 160°F (71.1°C), and fish 145°F (62.8°C).

Additional Measures:

Refrigeration and Storage: Refrigerate perishable foods promptly, preferably within two hours of purchase or preparation. Keep the refrigerator temperature at or below 40°F (4.4°C). Store leftovers in airtight containers and consume them within a safe timeframe to avoid bacterial growth.

Educate Household Members: Ensure everyone in the household is aware of these hygiene and food safety practices. Teach children the importance of handwashing and safe food handling to instill healthy habits from a young age.

By diligently following these measures, you can significantly reduce the risk of Salmonella transmission within your household. Prevention starts with simple yet effective practices that focus on cleanliness, separation, and safe food handling. These habits not only protect you and your family but also contribute to overall food safety and well-being.

Preventing further spread within the household.

Preventing the spread of Salmonella within your household is crucial to safeguard the health of your family members and prevent potential outbreaks. Here's an in-depth look at effective measures to stem the transmission of this harmful bacterium:

Rigorous Hand Hygiene:

Frequent and Thorough Handwashing: Make handwashing a steadfast habit, especially at critical times like before handling food, after using the restroom, changing diapers, or caring for someone who is ill. Scrub your hands vigorously with soap and water for at least 20 seconds, ensuring you clean between your fingers and under your nails.

Rigorous Surface Disinfection:

Regular Cleaning and Disinfecting: Consistently clean and disinfect surfaces that frequently encounter food or might come into contact with harmful bacteria. Focus on areas like countertops, cutting boards, knives, and kitchen utensils. Use hot, soapy water to scrub these surfaces thoroughly, followed by a disinfectant or a diluted bleach solution to ensure proper sanitation.

Safe Food Handling Practices:

Separation of Raw and Ready-to-Eat Foods: Take care to separate raw foods, such as raw meat, poultry, or seafood, from ready-to-eat foods like fruits, vegetables, and cooked items. Use separate cutting boards and utensils for raw and cooked foods to prevent cross-contamination.

Proper Cooking Temperatures: Ensure that foods, especially meat products, are cooked to safe internal temperatures. Utilize a food thermometer to accurately gauge the internal temperature of meats. For instance, cook poultry to an internal temperature of 165°F (73.9°C), ground beef to 160°F (71.1°C), and fish to 145°F (62.8°C) to eliminate harmful bacteria like Salmonella.

Additional Preventive Measures:

Prompt Refrigeration and Storage: Refrigerate perishable foods promptly, ideally within two hours of purchase or preparation. Maintain your refrigerator at a temperature of 40°F (4.4°C) or below to impede bacterial growth. Store leftovers in airtight containers and consume them within a safe timeframe.

Educating Household Members: Foster an environment of awareness and responsibility within your household. Educate all members, including children, about proper handwashing techniques and the significance of safe food handling. Encourage them to adopt these practices as a routine part of their daily activities.

Responding swiftly to suspected exposure to Salmonella is key to preventing further illness and safeguarding others. Taking proactive measures, seeking medical guidance when necessary, and maintaining meticulous hygiene practices within the household not only aid in personal recovery but also prevent the spread of illness to those around you. Remember, staying informed and acting promptly is crucial in dealing with suspected exposure to Salmonella.

Chapter 8

Preventive Measures and Guidelines

Hygiene and Handwashing: Emphasize regular handwashing, especially before handling food, after using the restroom, touching animals, or engaging in outdoor activities. Proper hand hygiene is a powerful preventive tool against Salmonella.

Safe Food Handling: Practice caution when handling and preparing food. Use separate cutting boards and utensils for raw and cooked foods. Ensure meats are cooked thoroughly to safe temperatures. Refrigerate perishable items promptly.

Proper Produce Handling: Wash fruits and vegetables thoroughly under running water, even if you're planning to peel them. This minimizes the risk of bacteria transferring from the surface to the flesh when cutting or peeling.

Food Safety Guidelines for Consumers:

Be Aware of High-Risk Foods: Understand which foods are more prone to Salmonella contamination, such as raw or undercooked eggs, poultry, unpasteurized milk, and raw fruits and vegetables.

Safe Shopping and Storage: When grocery shopping, keep raw meats separate from other foods in your cart and use separate bags for raw meats. Store raw meats on the bottom shelf of the refrigerator to prevent juices from dripping onto other foods.

Follow Expiry Dates and Storage Instructions: Pay attention to expiration dates on food packaging. Follow storage instructions and refrigerate perishable items promptly after purchase to maintain freshness and prevent bacterial growth.

Avoiding Consumption of Recalled Products:

Stay Updated with Recalls: Stay informed about food recalls by regularly checking recall notices or alerts issued by the Food and Drug Administration (FDA) or other relevant authorities. Immediately discard or return any recalled products.

Check Product Labels: Read product labels thoroughly to verify if a particular food item has been recalled. If uncertain, contact the manufacturer or retailer for clarification before consuming the product.

Educating About Proper Handling and Storage of Produce:

Education and Awareness: Educate individuals, especially in households with vulnerable members like children or the elderly, about the importance of proper food handling and storage practices to prevent Salmonella contamination.

Proper Refrigeration and Cooking: Stress the significance of refrigerating perishable items promptly and cooking food items thoroughly. Teach proper techniques for washing and handling fresh produce to mitigate the risk of contamination.

By proactively adopting these preventive measures, adhering to food safety guidelines, staying informed about recalls, and educating others, individuals can significantly reduce the risk of Salmonella contamination and infection, ensuring a safer and healthier environment for themselves and their communities.

Chapter 9

Collaborative Efforts and Solutions

The Cantaloupe Salmonella Outbreak has highlighted the importance of collaborative efforts and solutions in outbreak investigation and prevention. In this chapter, we'll explore the role of CDC, FDA, and other partners in outbreak investigation and prevention, collaborative strategies and initiatives to tackle future outbreaks, innovations in food safety technology and regulations, and success stories and lessons learned from past outbreaks.

Role of CDC, FDA, and Other Partners in Outbreak Investigation and Prevention

The Centers for Disease Control and Prevention (CDC) and the Food and Drug Administration (FDA) play a critical role in outbreak investigation and prevention. The CDC is responsible for monitoring and detecting outbreaks of foodborne illness, while the FDA is responsible for regulating the safety of food products. Both agencies work closely with state and local health departments to investigate outbreaks and identify the source of contamination.

In addition to the CDC and FDA, other partners involved in outbreak investigation and prevention include state and local health departments, regulatory agencies, food industry partners, and academic institutions. These partners work together to identify the source of contamination, prevent the spread of illness, and develop strategies to improve food safety.

Collaborative Strategies and Initiatives to Tackle Future Outbreaks

Collaborative strategies and initiatives are essential to tackling future outbreaks of foodborne illness. One such initiative is the New Era of Smarter Food Safety, which was launched by the FDA in 2020. The New Era of Smarter Food Safety is a blueprint for improving the safety of the food supply chain by leveraging technology and other tools to create a more digital, traceable food system.

Other collaborative strategies and initiatives include the use of whole genome sequencing to identify the source of contamination, the development of new technologies to improve food safety, and the implementation of new regulations to prevent contamination. By working together, public health officials, regulatory agencies, and food industry partners can develop effective strategies to prevent future outbreaks of foodborne illness.

Innovations in Food Safety Technology and Regulations

Innovations in food safety technology and regulations are critical to preventing future outbreaks of foodborne illness. One such innovation is the use of whole genome sequencing to identify the source of contamination. Whole genome sequencing allows public health officials to identify the specific strain of bacteria responsible for an outbreak, which can help identify the source of contamination and prevent future outbreaks.

Other innovations in food safety technology include the use of blockchain to improve traceability in the food supply chain, the development of new packaging materials to prevent contamination, and the use of artificial intelligence to identify potential sources of contamination. In addition to technological innovations, new regulations are also being implemented to prevent contamination, such as the Food Safety Modernization Act (FSMA).

Success Stories and Lessons Learned from Past Outbreaks.

Past outbreaks of foodborne illness have provided valuable lessons for preventing future outbreaks. For example, the 2002-2003 SARS epidemic in Hong Kong left a lasting impact on the region's public health system, leading to the adoption of a clearly defined, tiered command structure to prepare for and respond to future outbreaks 3. Similarly, the 2014 Ebola outbreak in West Africa highlighted the importance of community-based health systems in responding quickly and effectively to epidemics.

Collaborative efforts and solutions are essential to preventing future outbreaks of foodborne illness. By working together, public health officials, regulatory agencies, and food industry partners can develop effective strategies to identify the source of contamination, prevent the spread of illness, and improve food safety.

Chapter 10

The World of Cantaloupes

Cantaloupes are a type of muskmelon that is widely enjoyed around the world. In this chapter, we'll explore the origin, history, and nutritional value of cantaloupes, the different types and varieties of cantaloupes, the cultivation, harvesting, and distribution of cantaloupes, and the culinary uses and benefits of cantaloupes beyond the outbreak context.

Understanding cantaloupes

Geographical Origins:

Cantaloupes, scientifically known as Cucumis melo var. cantalupensis, are believed to trace their roots to the historical region encompassing Iran, India, and parts of Africa. These regions are considered the cradle of cultivation for this delectable fruit.

Centuries of Cultivation and Cultural Heritage:

The cultivation of cantaloupes spans centuries, entwining with the rich tapestry of cultural history. In ancient times, these succulent fruits held a symbolic significance, often representing fertility, abundance, and indulgence. Their prominence extended beyond mere sustenance—they were revered, depicted in artworks, and incorporated into ceremonial rituals, highlighting their cultural and spiritual significance.

Nutritional Value of Cantaloupes:

Vitamins and Minerals: Cantaloupes boast an impressive nutritional profile. They are a treasure trove of essential vitamins, prominently featuring vitamins A and C. Vitamin A, in the form of beta-carotene, contributes to eye health and supports the immune system. Vitamin C acts as a potent antioxidant, aiding in cell protection and immune function. Additionally, these fruits offer a good dose of dietary fiber and potassium, vital for heart health and digestive wellness.

Low-Calorie and Antioxidant-Rich: Remarkably, cantaloupes offer this nutritional bounty while being exceptionally low in calories, making them an ideal choice for those mindful of their calorie intake. With merely 60 calories in a 1-cup serving, they serve as a guilt-free, delectable snack option. Moreover, their richness in antioxidants, including beta-carotene and vitamin C, bestows them with the power to combat cell damage and potentially lower the risk of chronic diseases, presenting a flavorful way to fortify your health.

Culinary Appeal and Versatility:

Delightful Taste and Versatility: Apart from their nutritional prowess, cantaloupes entice with their sweet, refreshing taste and versatile culinary uses. They're a delightful addition to fruit salads, smoothies, or enjoyed simply sliced and savored on a sunny day. Their juicy, aromatic flesh adds a burst of flavor to both sweet and savory dishes, exemplifying their versatility in culinary creations.

Understanding the origins, historical significance, and nutritional richness of cantaloupes not only enhances appreciation for this luscious fruit but also illuminates its multifaceted value—be it as a cultural symbol, a nutritional powerhouse, or a versatile culinary delight that graces our tables through the ages.

Different types and varieties of cantaloupes

North American Cantaloupe (Cucumis melo 'Reticulatus')
The quintessential grocery store variety, this classic cantaloupe boasts a textured, netted rind and vibrant orange flesh. Widely recognized for its sweet taste and juiciness, it's a go-to choice for many due to its familiar appearance and delightful flavor.

European Cantaloupe (Cucumis melo 'Cantalupensis')
Distinguished by its light green, ridged skin, the European variety bears little resemblance to its North American counterpart. Renowned for its unique appearance, this type offers a distinct taste and texture, making it a sought-after option in regions favoring its cultivation.

Asian Cantaloupe (Cucumis melo 'Oriental Sweet')
Celebrated for its exceptional sweetness, the Asian cantaloupe boasts soft, orange-hued flesh that delivers a luscious, juicy flavor. Its popularity stems from its delectable taste and texture, making it a prized choice among fruit enthusiasts.

French Cantaloupe (Cucumis melo 'Charentais')
This variety is revered for its exquisite sweetness and aromatic fragrance. Often incorporated into desserts due to its exceptional taste, the French cantaloupe captivates with its delicate flavor profile and alluring scent, making it a preferred option for culinary indulgence.

Galia Cantaloupe (Cucumis melo 'Galia')
With its greenish-yellow skin and sweet, succulent flesh, the Galia cantaloupe stands out for its distinctive appearance and delectable taste. Its juicy texture and subtle sweetness make it a popular choice, offering a delightful addition to fruit salads or a refreshing standalone treat.

Factors Influencing Varieties

Soil Type, Climate, and Geographic Location: The choice of cantaloupe varieties is influenced by diverse environmental factors. Soil type, climatic conditions, and geographic location play pivotal roles in determining which varieties thrive best in specific regions. Varieties are often cultivated based on these factors, ensuring optimal growth and yield.

Culinary Diversity and Preferences

Culinary Applications: Each variety of cantaloupe brings a unique flavor profile and texture, allowing for a diverse range of culinary applications. From fresh consumption to culinary creations, these varieties offer a spectrum of tastes and characteristics, catering to a myriad of preferences and culinary adventures.

The array of cantaloupe varieties, each with its distinctive appearance, taste, and culinary applications, exemplifies the diversity and richness of this beloved fruit. Whether relishing the familiar sweetness of the North American type or savoring the unique flavors of the European, Asian, French, or Galia varieties, exploring these diverse options adds depth and richness to the world of culinary delights.

Cultivation, harvesting, and distribution of cantaloupes

Ideal Growing Conditions

Cantaloupes thrive in warm, sunny climates with ample sunlight and well-draining soil. They require a sufficient supply of water and nutrients, often necessitating soil enriched with organic matter for optimal growth. Cultivation practices involve careful monitoring of temperature, moisture levels, and soil quality to ensure robust growth.

Planting and Growth Cycle

Cantaloupes are typically planted in spring after the threat of frost has passed. The seeds are sown directly into the soil, allowing the plants to germinate and establish their root systems. As the vines grow, they require adequate spacing to sprawl and produce healthy fruits. Farmers monitor the growth, providing necessary irrigation and fertilization as the plants develop.

Harvesting Cantaloupes

Timing of Harvest: Cantaloupes are usually ready for harvest in late summer or early fall, varying slightly depending on the specific variety and growing conditions. Farmers assess several indicators to determine readiness, including the fruit's appearance, aroma, and texture.

Ripeness Indicators

A ripe cantaloupe exhibits specific signs: the fruit develops a distinct coloration (varying from green to beige or orange, depending on the variety), emits a sweet and fragrant aroma from the stem end, and the rind texture changes from hard to slightly yielding upon gentle pressure.

Harvesting Process

Selective Picking: Farmers hand-harvest cantaloupes individually, ensuring selective picking of fully ripe fruits. This process involves carefully detaching the fruit from the vine, preserving its integrity and quality.

Post-Harvest Handling

Once harvested, the cantaloupes undergo sorting and washing to remove debris or soil. This meticulous process ensures cleanliness and prepares the fruits for distribution and packaging.

Distribution to Retailers

Sorting and Packaging: The sorted cantaloupes are categorized based on quality and size before packaging. Packaging methods may vary, ranging from individual wrapping to bulk containers, safeguarding the fruits during transit.

Distribution to Market

After packaging, the cantaloupes are transported to distribution centers and subsequently delivered to grocery stores and other retailers. Ensuring freshness and quality, these fruits make their way to consumers, ready to delight palates with their sweetness and flavor.

From the careful cultivation and attentive nurturing of cantaloupe plants through the growth cycle to the meticulous harvesting and post-harvest handling, each step in the process contributes to delivering fresh, ripe, and flavorful fruits to consumers. The cultivation, harvesting, and distribution of cantaloupes entail a comprehensive journey that showcases the dedication of farmers and ensures the availability of this beloved fruit in markets for everyone to enjoy.

Culinary uses and benefits beyond the outbreak context.

Fresh Consumption and Salads

Cantaloupes are a delightful choice for fresh consumption due to their juicy, sweet flesh. Sliced or cubed, they make a refreshing snack on hot days or a juicy addition to fruit salads, adding a burst of flavor and texture to the ensemble.

Smoothies and Beverages

Their naturally sweet taste and high water content make cantaloupes a fantastic ingredient for smoothies and beverages. Blended with other fruits or yogurt, they contribute a luscious, fruity essence to smoothie concoctions or refreshing drinks.

Dessert and Culinary Creativity

Cantaloupes elevate desserts with their sweet profile. They can serve as a topping for ice creams, sorbets, or yogurt parfaits, imparting a refreshing note to these treats. Additionally, their versatility shines in creative culinary experiments—they can be incorporated into cakes, tarts, or popsicles for a unique twist.

Cooking Methods for Unique Flavors

Surprisingly, cantaloupes exhibit delightful flavors when exposed to heat. Grilling, roasting, or baking these fruits can unlock their natural sweetness, caramelizing their sugars and intensifying their taste. This brings out unique flavor profiles, adding depth to savory dishes or providing a sweet counterbalance in various recipes.

Health Benefits Beyond Culinary Pleasure

Nutritional Powerhouse

Beyond their culinary allure, cantaloupes offer a treasure trove of health benefits. They are rich in vitamins A and C, antioxidants, dietary fiber, and potassium. These nutrients bolster immunity, support vision health, aid digestion, and promote heart health.

Hydration and Wellness

Cantaloupes, with their high water content, contribute to hydration, especially during hot weather. They offer a hydrating snack option while providing essential vitamins and minerals, ensuring overall well-being.

Low-Calorie, Nutrient-Rich Choice

Remarkably, cantaloupes offer all these health benefits while being low in calories. With only about 60 calories per cup, they provide a satisfying, nutrient-rich option for those watching their calorie intake.

The culinary potential of cantaloupes transcends traditional boundaries, offering a spectrum of culinary delights from fresh snacks to gourmet creations. Beyond their delicious taste and culinary versatility, cantaloupes contribute significantly to health and wellness, making them a beloved choice not just during outbreaks but as a versatile, nutritious, and refreshing addition to everyday meals and culinary creations.

Conclusion

Through the exploration of the Cantaloupe Salmonella Outbreak and the multifaceted facets surrounding cantaloupes, this book has provided a comprehensive insight into the complexities of food safety, public health, and the rich world of this beloved fruit. From understanding the origins of the outbreak to delving into the nuances of Salmonella poisoning and preventive measures, each chapter has unraveled critical details.

We ventured into the realms of microbiology, learning about Salmonella bacteria, their behavior, and the myriad strains that pose health risks. We navigated through the historical tapestry of cantaloupes, uncovering their origins, cultural significance, and nutritional bounty beyond their delectable taste.

Exploring the cultivation, harvesting, and distribution unveiled the meticulous journey from farm to table, underscoring the dedication of growers and ensuring the supply of fresh, flavorful cantaloupes. Furthermore, our culinary odyssey showcased the versatile uses of cantaloupes, extending beyond salads and snacks to delightful desserts, smoothies, and savory culinary experiments.

The narrative didn't merely revolve around an outbreak but opened doors to broader discussions on food safety, nutrition, and wellness, underscoring the significance of proper handling, hygiene, and informed consumer choices. Each chapter painted a comprehensive picture, blending scientific insights with practical guidance, empowering readers to make informed decisions regarding their health and dietary choices.

As we conclude this journey, let us carry forward this amalgamation of knowledge and awareness. Let's embrace the importance of food safety, celebrate the versatility of cantaloupes in our kitchens, and continue fostering a culture of well-being and informed choices. May this book serve as a beacon, enlightening minds and nurturing healthier, safer communities for years to come.